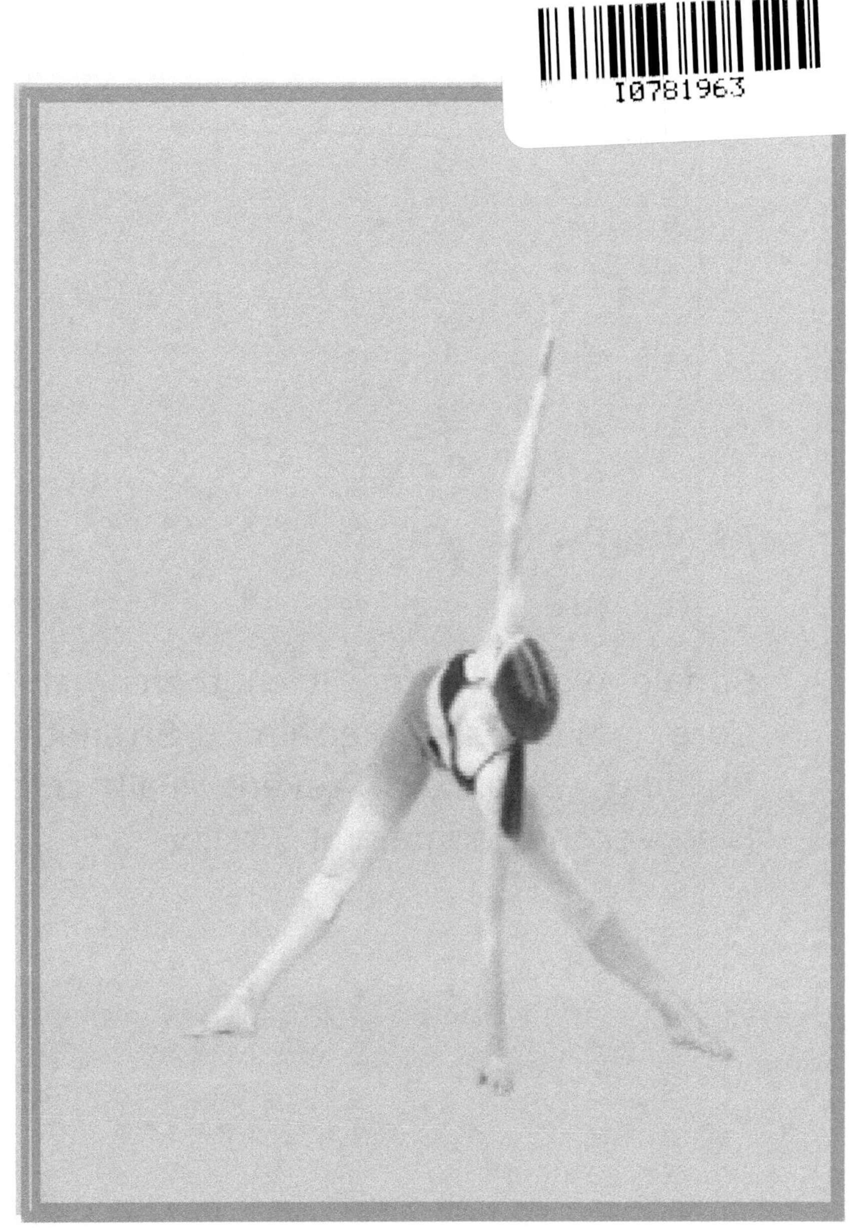

40 CORE EXERCISES FOR SENIORS OVER 50

Simple Workouts for Strengthening the Core Muscles, Reclaim Strength, Building Balance, Prevent Fall and Discover the Fountain of Vitality.

PAUL KELVIN

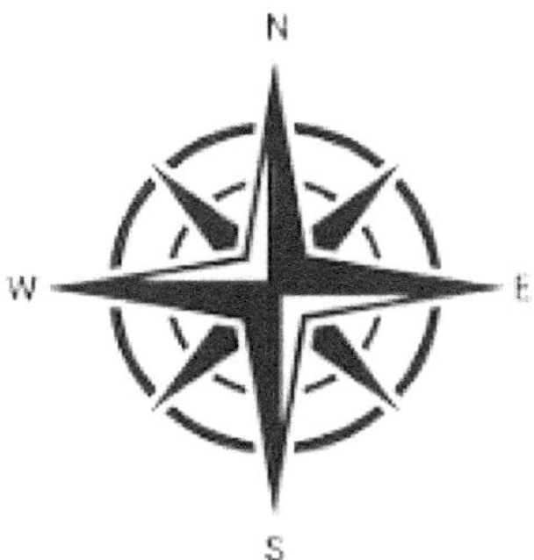

TABLE OF CONTENTS

CHAPTER 4: CORE YOGA POSES TO IMPROVE CORE FLEXIBILITY AND MOBILITY..57

CHAPTER FIVE: PILATE WORKOUTS TO IMPROVE CORE STABILITY AND BALANCE AND

INTRODUCTION

With "40 Core Workouts for Seniors over 50', you will explore the fountain of Vitality," this book will help you to take a close look at our cherished older community's physical health and well-being.

This detailed book demonstrates our steadfast dedication to assisting seniors in realizing their full potential and enjoying life to the fullest.

These pages provide a wealth of carefully chosen core workouts that have been tailored to fit the special requirements and capabilities of elderly citizens. We know that having a strong core is essential for general stability, balance, and mobility—all of which are critical for leading an independent and active life.

However, this book offers much more than just a list of workouts. It is a guide for improving your health and regaining your excitement for life. Whether you are spending time with your grandkids, we think that becoming older shouldn't stop you from doing the things you love.

You will feel renewed when you are full of strength, resilience, and confidence by adding these specifically created core workouts into your daily routine. This will enable you to fully enjoy every moment of your life.

Every workout routine in this book has been thoughtfully designed with your safety and well-being in mind. You'll be led through a progressive program that progressively increases your core strength while taking into account any current restrictions or health issues.

The instructions are step-by-step and are supported by a few comprehensive pictures.

However, this book covers more than simply physical health. It explores the significance of self-care and mentality, acknowledging that genuine vitality involves more than simply the physical body.

"Core Workouts for Seniors over 50 is a road toward transformation, not just a guide. It proves our point that no matter how many years have gone, age is just a number and you can still influence your future.

Now, flip through these pages, welcome the knowledge they contain, and set off on an incredible journey that will transform your idea of what it is to grow old with grace and experience life to the fullest.

CHAPTER 1: EMBRACING THE POWER OF A STRONG CORE, IMPROVING CORE STRENGTH AND VITALITY

The set of muscles such as in the midsection of the human body that support your spine, pelvis, hips, lower back, abs, and stomach. It is referred to as your body's core. The body's core is made up of numerous muscles and muscle groups.

Our core can move in all three planes of motion and has a three-dimensional depth. The majority of the muscles are concealed beneath the surface muscles that individuals usually train.

The transverse abdominals, multifidus, diaphragm, pelvic floor, and several deeper muscles are examples of the deeper muscles.

IMPORTANCE OF THE CORE TO THE HUMAN BODY:

The core muscles play an important role in the human body. Some of them are:

First, we understand that there are two primary purposes for the core muscles.

- to transfer force from the lower body to the upper body and vice versa;
- to protect the spine from an excessive load.

It is important to keep in mind that our ability to perform at our best and avoid injuries is enhanced by having a strong, stable core.

Spinal injuries usually result from a combination of forward bending, sideways bending, or excessive rotation. Back injuries are more often related to a history of high load and poor mechanics than to a single incidence (lifting something heavy).

Ideally, according to research, we should build 360 degrees of strength around the spine to protect it as we move, run, leap, toss, lift items, and transfer force throughout our body. When every muscle in our torso, shoulders, and hips functions as a unit, we do this.

Keep in mind that building a stronger core with exercises helps a senior to improve their health and enable them to stay younger and more active in their daily life activity.

CORE STRENGTH:

The ability of your torso and pelvic muscles to function as a unit to stabilize, balance, and support your spine and complete body is known as core strength.

The muscles of the core consist of the abdominals, the obliques (side abdominals), the pelvic floor, the lower back, and deep stabilizing muscles like the multifidus and transverse abdominis.

Maintaining good posture, doing daily tasks with ease, and engaging in physical activities or sports all depend on having a strong core. It facilitates smooth force transfer between the upper and lower bodies and acts as a base for movement.

A robust core can improve physical health overall, lower the chance of injury, and improve sports performance.

For example, the muscles in your core are essential for bending, twisting, lifting, and reaching. They provide the spine support, maintaining its correct alignment and protection. Furthermore, a strong core can strengthen functional movements needed for daily chores, improve balance and coordination, and reduce back discomfort.

Having well-defined abdominal muscles is just one aspect of core strength; another is having a coordinated, balanced, and harmoniously functioning collection of muscles.

A healthy core integrates the deep stabilizing muscles with the surface muscles, forming a strong and durable base for the body's mobility and stability.

BENEFITS OF EXERCISES TO THE CORE MUSCLES:

Combining workouts that focus on the various muscle groups in the core is necessary to build core strength.

Planks, bridges, rotational exercises, and functional movements—movements that work the core while carrying out tasks like lifting weights, walking, or playing sports can all be included in this set of exercises.

It's crucial to remember that building appropriate posture, body awareness, and muscular endurance are all aspects of improving core strength in addition to strength training.

Frequent core exercises can enhance core strength, stability, and general physical when paired with a well-rounded fitness program and a healthy lifestyle.

However, we are going to delve into the various exercises that will help to strengthen and keep the core muscles healthy in the remaining chapters of this book.

But before we start, each exercise in this book, you need to ensure that you do not have any form of injury or sickness, if you do please consult your healthcare provider before attempting any of these exercises.

It is also important to keep in mind that all the exercises in this book can be done at home whether you have any equipment or not, you don't need to go to any gym house or hire any coach just create a space in your house, grab a mat, chair and maybe a towel or pillow for support then you are good to start.

Finally, This book is well-packaged in a simple way that the exercises are well-explained and easy to understand with step-by-step instructional guides.

CHAPTER 2: GENTLE CORE STRENGTHENING EXERCISES FOR SENIORS WITH LIMITED MOBILITY AND FITNESS LEVEL

In this chapter, we are going to start with simple exercises for seniors who have limited mobility and strength. The following are the exercises:

BIRD DOG STRETCH:

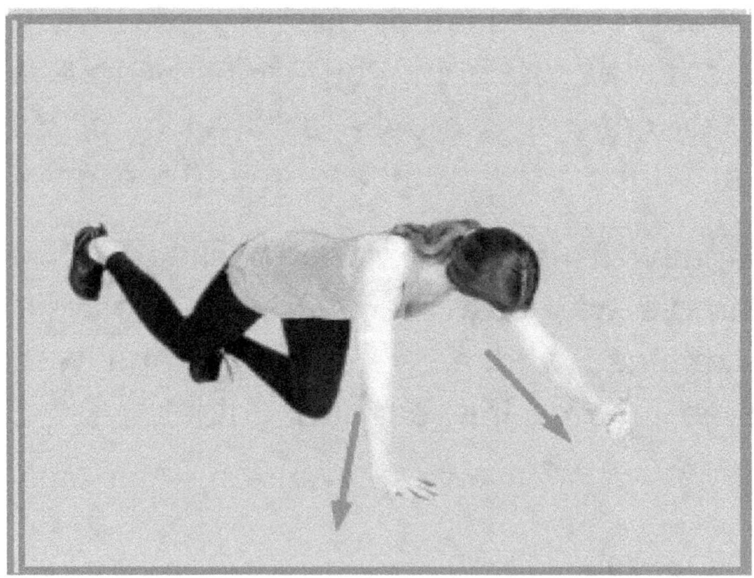

This stretch targets the whole body for an increased range of motion. It helps to strengthen the core, back muscles, and hips relieve lower back pain, and improve proper posture.

You will need an exercise mat for this activity. For additional padding, place a folded towel or flat pillow beneath your knees. A mirror may be used to verify your alignment.

For this exercise to be effective the following are the steps to take:

- Start in the tabletop posture on all fours.
- Put your hands under your shoulders and your knees beneath your hips.
- Make sure your abs are working to keep your spine neutral.
- Press the blades of your shoulder together.

- Maintaining your shoulders and hips parallel to the floor, raise your left leg and right arm.
- To look down at the floor, drop your chin toward your chest and lengthen the back of your neck.
- After a little while, hold this position and then return to the beginning position.
- Raise your right leg and left arm, and stay in this posture for a little while.
- Go back to the initial position. this is a round.
- Do two to three sets of eight to twelve reps.
- appropriate method and alignment

GLUTE BRIDGE EXERCISE:

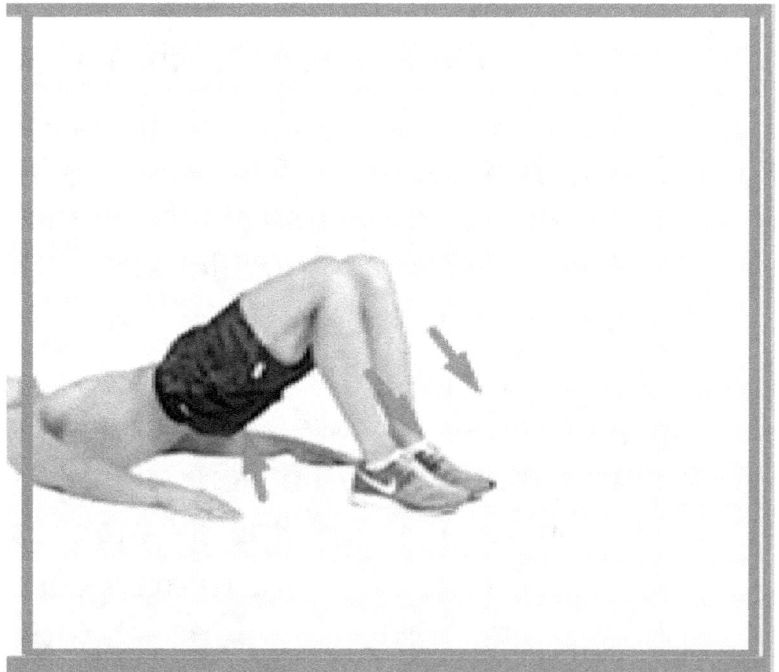

This workout helps to strengthen the core muscles and keep them strong and healthy.

The following are the instructions to follow when performing this exercise:

- To begin this exercise, put your feet flat on the floor and your knees bent, and lie down on your back with your knees about shoulder-width apart. Ensure that your heels are 6–8 inches away from your glutes and that your toes are pointed straight ahead. Spread your arms out flat on both sides, opening your palms to the sky.

- Squeeze your core, tighten your glutes, and slowly lift your hips.
- As you raise your hips as high as you can, take care not to arch your back. A proper glute bridge consists of lifting your hips till your torso produces a straight line from your shoulder up to your knee.
- As soon as you get to the top of the glute bridge, clench your glutes and hold the position for a short while.
- With controlled movement, return your hips to the floor while

maintaining the tension in your glutes and abs.

LYING DOWN LEG LIFT EXERCISE:

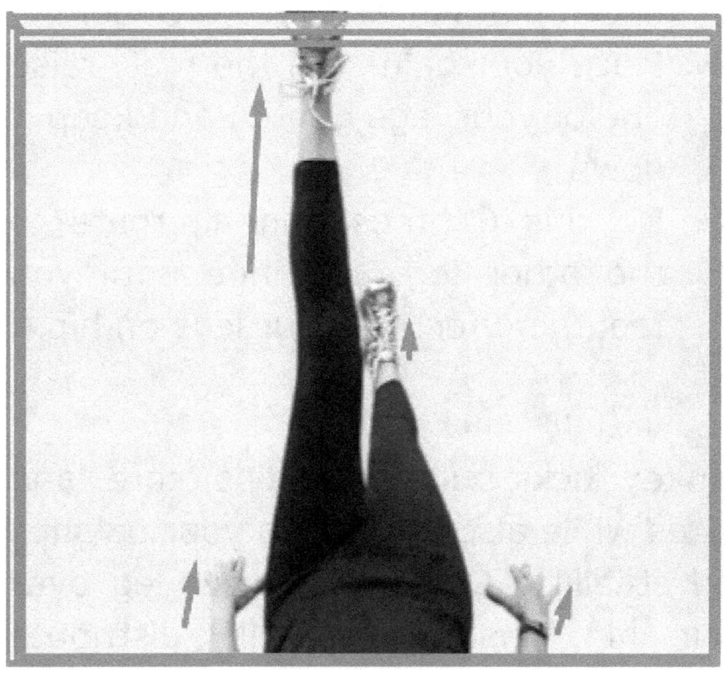

This exercise has almost the same effect as the seated leg lift exercise. It is also called the range of motion exercise. It helps to strengthen the hips, the legs, and the upper body muscles. The following are the guides to performing this effectively;

- First, lie down straight with your back on a mat and face the roof.
- Place your palms on the mat, raise one of your legs gently, and keep it down.
- Do this 6 times and alternate to the other leg. Continue until you feel the effect on your legs on hip.

DONKEY KICK EXERCISE:

Donkey kicks build your hips, core, and glutes while also improving your balance and stability. Don't raise your leg over your hip; instead, equally distribute your weight.

The following is the step-by-step guide to do this exercise:

- To start this exercise, grab a mat and spread it on the floor.

- Next, kneel with both knees your both then spread your palms on the mat, and then flex one knee deeper to lift your foot slightly off the floor.
- freeze the knee in this position then dorsiflex the ankle.
- Exhale and extend at the hips to lift that leg until your quad forms a symmetrical extension of your torso.
- ensure that you do not lift the thigh higher than the torso as this could cause compression disc in the lower back.
- inhale flex at the hip then draw the leg back.
- Perform the several repetitions that you can and alternate to the other leg.

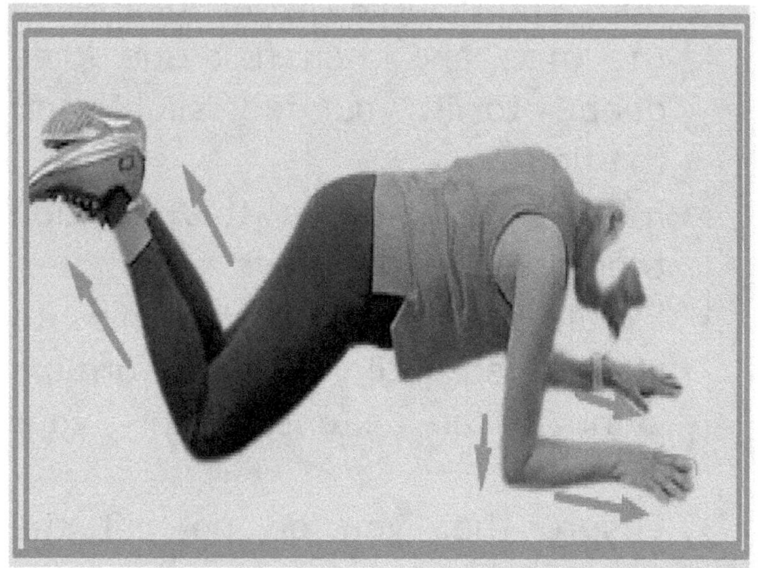

This exercise helps to improve overall core strength. It usually targets each of the core muscles at the same time if you hold onto the ground.

With its seemingly simple form, the plank can be one of the easiest workouts for your core, but it can also be one of the most taxing ones. Despite the difficulty, the workout's full-body effect will work your core with excellent benefit.

To do the plank exercise follow the instructions below:

- Be on your knees on a mat, and shift your weight so that you will be basically on the tissue above your knees.
- Your shoulder should be in alignment with your wrist then hold it for a few seconds, place your shoulder underneath your shoulders, and hold for a second. Do this exercise as long as you can, if you are tired you can rest.

WALL PLANK EXERCISE:

This exercise is almost the same as the floor plank exercise.

Follow the instructions below and carry out the exercise:

- To start this exercise against the wall, place your forearms.
- Take a small step backwards to make your entire body slightly angled.
- Maintain a straight spine and hip alignment.
- Ensure that your feet remain flat as well.
- Hold the position.
- Take care to step away from the wall.

CHAPTER 3: BEST-SEATED CORE EXERCISES TO ENHANCE STABILITY AND STRENGTH

In this chapter, we are going to practice the seated exercises that can help to improve strength and stability.

Research has proven that as we get older, the body tends to get weaker by the day, this is the reason it is important to engage in profitable exercises that will help to build up weak muscles in the body.

These exercises are very good for seniors because they don't have to go through the stress of standing only what they need to do to participate in these exercises, grab a chair sit and start the exercises.

The following are the different core seated exercises that can improve strength:

SEATED LEG LIFT EXERCISE:

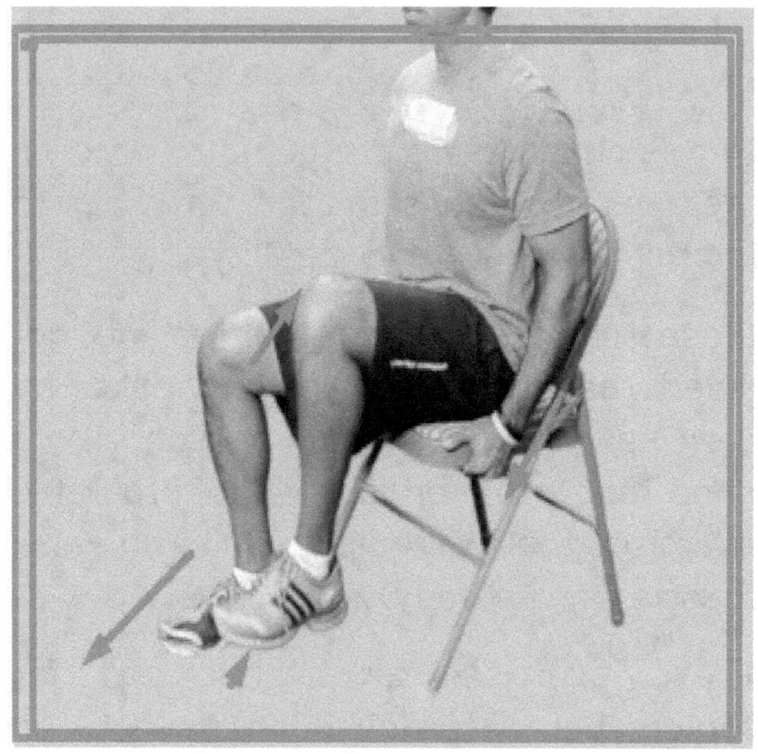

Leg lifts are a fantastic method to simultaneously engage your oblique muscles and abs.

Additionally, you can carry out these exercises in a seated or lying down position, based on your preference.

The following are the guides to performing this exercise:

- Begin this exercise, by sitting straight on a sturdy chair, your arms should be positioned by your side. Then bend your knees and feet flat on the floor.
- Maintaining the beginning position for your opposing leg, raise one leg while using your core. maintain a straight back.
- Keep your posture for three seconds. After you've taken a step back, repeat with the other leg.
- As many repetitions as you can, switch up your legs. Always remember to take baby steps and work your way up.

SEATED HALF ROLL-BACK EXERCISE:

This exercise is also known as a core-strengthening exercise. It helps to strengthen your abdominal and upper back muscles with the following guides:

- Sit straight at the edge of a sturdy chair, then bend your knees and your feet flat on the floor.
- Ensure you move your arms out in front of your chest, make a circle, and keep your back in a straight position.
- Dip your face toward the arm circle while rolling onto your back. It might be compared to scooping your abdominal area.
- Once you've reached your limit, tense your abs and slowly return to your initial upright position.
- Be on your knees on a mat, and shift your weight so that you will be basically on the tissue above your knees.
- Your shoulder should be in alignment with your wrist then hold

it for a few seconds, place your shoulder underneath your shoulders, and hold for a second. Do this exercise as long as you can, if you are tired you can rest.

SEATED SIDE BENDS:

Senior core exercises don't always need lying down. A basic, well-made chair may open up a world of other workouts. Your internal and external obliques, as well as your abdominal muscles, are formed by the sitting side bends.

- Take a seat on your chair and do the following movements to perform the sitting side bends:
- Lay your feet flat on the ground and bend your knees.
- With your elbow pulled out to line it with your ear, place the palm of your right hand on the back of your head. Keep your left arm dangling

over to the side while keeping it in line with your upper torso.

- Maintain a straight posture. Avoid hunching over or reclining.
- Inhale, then exhale and bend your body to the left, bringing your left arm closer to the floor.
- Pull your right elbow back as you lean. You'll experience a stretch on that side as a result.
- Inhale once more and return to the beginning position.
- After you've completed as many repetitions as you can, switch to the opposite arm.

SEATED DEAD BUG EXERCISE:

This exercise can help you work the muscles in your upper and lower abdomen.

- To do the dead bug, choose a sturdy chair that allows you to recline while maintaining a straight back and extended arms. It will work just as well with a basic fold-up chair. Then, adhere to these guidelines.

- Reposition yourself in the chair so that your back is straight.
- Keep your head up, contract your core, and simultaneously extend your left leg and raise your right arm.
- Keep your position for a moment.
- Go back to where you were before.
- Replicate the actions using different arms and legs.
- You should attempt the same when your core strength improves without the chair.

The steps would then be the same, but instead of using the chair's extra back support, you would sit on the floor, which would put more pressure on and improve your core muscles.

Alternatively, you may do the dead bug while lying down with your legs and arms in the air and your back on the ground. similar to this.

SEATED FORWARD ROLL-UP EXERCISE:

The sitting forward roll-up is a fantastic seated core exercise that is especially beneficial for seniors who are trying to target their upper and lower abdominal muscles.

- To start this exercise, sit in a sturdy chair, draw your feet back towards you, and stretch your legs so that your heels are on the floor.
- Align your arms with your legs so that they are out in front of you.

- After attempting to maintain the most appropriate, upright posture you are capable of, do the following:
- Inhale, roll your chin to your chest and maintain straight legs.
- Breathe out while your whole body bends toward your toes, following your chin.
- Breathe in and roll your body back when you are at your limit. Take your time and visualize each vertebrae rolling back one after the other.
- Repeat.

To get the most out of this workout, move gently. Make sure your shoulders and back don't give you any momentum since you want your abs to perform the heavy lifting.

Do not forget to roll the various body parts. Avoid launching them.

SEATED MARCHES:

This exercise helps the heart rate. Your thighs and hips will become more mobile and flexible after doing this workout.

The following are how to do this exercise:

- To start this exercise, towards the front of the chair take a seat.
- Keep your back straight, your feet hip-width apart, and your arms at your sides.
- To activate your core, contract the muscles in your abdomen.
- Keep your knee bent and raise your right leg as high as you can.
- Gradually bring your right foot down to the ground.
- To finish one rep, repeat the movement with your left leg.

- Perform two to three sets of ten to twelve repetitions.

SEATED JUMPING JACKS EXERCISE:

Shift to a full-body aerobic exercise by performing jumping jacks while seated. The traditional workout may improve coordination and mobility while also supporting heart and bone health.

How to do this exercise:

- Assume a forward-facing seat in your chair. Maintain a straight back, place your feet together, and keep your arms at your sides.
- To activate your core, bring your belly button in close to your spine.
- Step your legs apart approximately shoulder-width apart and raise your arms overhead.
- Step your feet together and bring your arms to your sides to revert to the beginning posture.

- Perform 10 to 12 repetitions as fast as you can.
- Finish two or three sets.

SIT-TO STANDS EXERCISE:

Your legs, hips, abs, and other core muscles are strengthened during the sit-to-stand exercise. It can also improve your balance and build muscle strength.

The following are the steps to performing this exercise:

- Place your hands on each side of your thighs as you take a seat closer to the front of the chair. Maintain a straight spine and space your feet hip-width apart.
- To activate your core, bring your belly button in close to your spine.
- By transferring your weight through your feet, lean forward from your hips.

- As you gently rise, take a breather and maintain your upright posture.
- To return to a sitting position, push your hips back and bend your knees.

SEATED ANKLE ABCS EXERCISE:

Increased ankle mobility from this exercise might help you walk more steadily on your feet. It serves as a strengthening and stretching workout as well.

The following are the steps to performing this exercise:

- Placing your feet flat on the floor and your palms on your thighs, assume a tall posture.
- Lift one leg straight out in front of you.
- Consider your great toe as a pen. Make the letters as large as you can as you write the alphabet with

your toe. Instead of moving your entire leg, move your foot.
- With your second leg, repeat movements 2 through 3 again.

You might try writing your name in cursive or spelling words backwards for an extra challenge if you can.

SEATED BEND FORWARD EXERCISES:

Your back muscles extend when you sit forward, which improves flexibility.

The following are how to do this exercise:

- With your feet shoulder-width apart, take a tall stance close to the edge of the chair.
- As you gradually bend forward from your hips, maintain a straight back.

- As you continue to bend forward, bring your chin into your lap and slide your hands down your calves.
- For ten to thirty seconds, hold the stretch.
- Straight up and gently to get back to the beginning.
- Three to five times, repeat.

SEATED CHEST STRETCHING EXERCISES

This sitting chest stretch may be used to start your relaxation routine; it can also improve your posture.

The following are the steps to take when performing this exercise:

- With your feet shoulder-width apart and your arms at your sides, take a tall stance or sit upright.
- With your palms pointing front, extend your arms out to your sides.

- Squeeze your shoulder blades together as you gently bring your arms back.
- After holding the stretch for ten to thirty seconds, go back to the initial position.
- Three to five times, repeat.

LEG CURLS WHILE STANDING:

This leg strengthener primarily targets your hamstrings and calves. Walking up and down stairs, for example, requires strong hamstrings.

They could also reduce the risk of injury and enhance athletic performance.

The following are the steps to take to carry out this exercise:

- Holding the back of the chair for balance, take a proud stance behind a strong chair.

- Switch to your left leg and contract your core.
- Bring your heel as near to your butt as possible as you bend your right knee. As you stand, make sure your leg is slightly bent and maintain your hip position.
- After a brief period of holding the curl, return your leg to its initial position.
- Perform twelve to fifteen repetitions.
- Apply the same pressure to your left knee.

CHAPTER 4: CORE EXERCISES FOR SENIORS TO BUILD STABILITY, BALANCE AND IMPROVE COORDINATION

In this chapter, we are going to learn how core exercises can help to improve balance and coordination for seniors.

In addition to helping you maintain good posture and avoid injuries, a strong and stable core is also very important for improving your general balance and coordination as a senior.

These exercises are specially designed to work the muscles involved in balance and coordination. Your ability to move with elegance, control, and stability will be enhanced by strengthening your core muscles and concentrating on good alignment.

The following are different balance and coordination exercises for seniors:

STANDING LEG SWING EXERCISE:

This exercise helps to strengthen the hamstring and the lower body.

The following is the step-by-step guide to perform this exercise:

- Stand straight with your legs hip-width apart and ensure that your hands should be by your sides.
- While keeping your balance and control, swing the opposing leg forward and backwards.
- Make ten to fifteen swings with each leg.
- You can swing your leg out to the side or do the swings with your eyes closed to make it more difficult.

WALL PUSH-UP EXERCISE:

The ability to perform push-ups with proper form is a strong indicator of your ability to withstand some of the effects of ageing.

Push-ups are an extremely important exercise for people as they age. They engage the muscle groups in the arms, chest, abdomen, hips, and legs providing a full-body workout with far-reaching benefits.

The following are the guides to performing this exercise:

- To start this exercise stand and face the wall with your feet shoulder-width apart.
- Place your both arms straight in front of you with your palm placed on the wall.
- Ensure you keep your stomach stuck straight on the back.

- Lean in and then press yourself off the wall.
- Repeat the process.
- Change how far your feet are from the wall. The exercise will be easier the closer you stand to the wall.

ROCK THE BOAT EXERCISE:

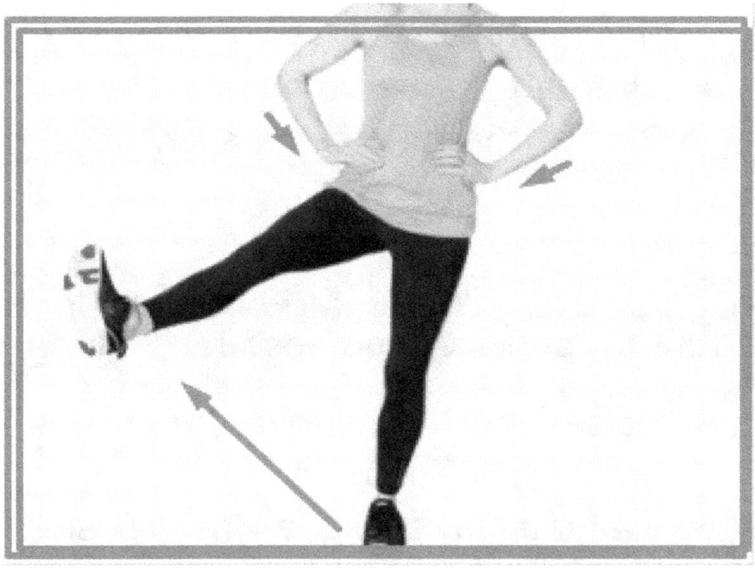

The following are the steps to carry out this exercise:

- Place your feet hip-distance apart as you stand.
- Raise your arms over your head and spread them apart.
- Raise your left foot off the ground and move your heel towards your buttocks by bending your knee.
- As long as 30 seconds, maintain this posture.
- alternate to the other side.
- Repeat three times on each side.

WALK ON A TIGHTROPE EXERCISE:

This easy workout enhances core strength, balance, and posture.

- Raise your arms over your head and spread them apart.
- Maintain a straight line of sight while keeping your eyes concentrated on a distant place.

- Take two to three seconds to pause each time you elevate your foot in this manner.
- Make 20 to 30 steps.

HEEL-TO-TOE STROLL EXERCISE:

This workout enhances balance and builds leg strength.

To perform this exercise do the following:

- Place your heels on the wall while you stand there.
- The left foot should be placed in front of the right foot.
- Put your right toes and left heel together.
- Next, align your right foot with your left foot.
- Connect your left toe with your right heel.
- Go through 20 steps further.

THE FLAMINGO STAND EXERCISE:

This exercise helps to strengthen the lower parts of the body.

Do the following to perform the exercise:

- Turn to stand on your right foot.
- Raise your left foot and kick your leg out in front of you.
- Keep your posture for ten to fifteen seconds.
- By extending your hands toward your outstretched foot, you may make it harder.
- Shake out your legs and go back to where you were.
- Do this three times.
- alternate and perform the activity on the other side.

TIA CHI CLOUD HANDS:

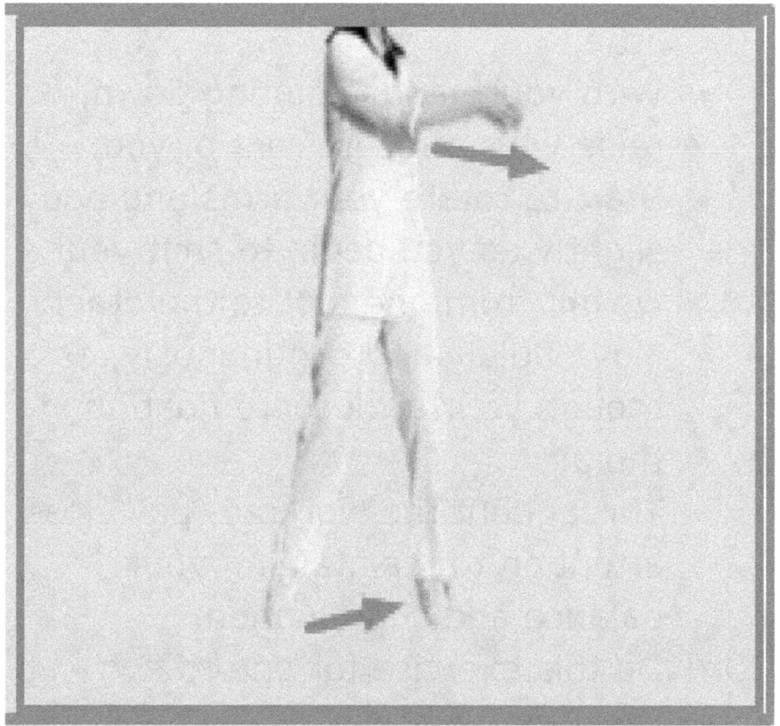

This exercise helps to strengthen the core muscles and improve balance:

The following is how to do the exercise:

- Place your feet shoulder-width apart and flex your knees just a little.
- With your hands pointing down, raise your arms in front of you.
- Start to rotate your arms and body slightly as you begin to shift your weight from one foot to the other.
- Move fluidly and continuously, as though your arms were floating in the air.
- Throughout the workout, pay close attention to maintaining your balance and coordination.
- Do this exercise for one to two minutes.

CHAPTER 5: CORE YOGA POSES TO IMPROVE CORE FLEXIBILITY AND MOBILITY

Yoga poses are very easy to perform. They are used for improving the overall core strength.

However, in this chapter, we will participate in the various yoga poses that will help to improve the overall core strength of all the body parts.

The following are the different yoga poses:

TREE POSES EXERCISE:

This exercise helps to strengthen the core and improve balance and stability.

When performing this exercise ensure that you do not place your foot on your knee.

The following are the steps to take when performing this exercise:

- To begin this exercise, stand up straight, and ensure you move your weight to your right foot.
- Place the sole of your foot on your thigh, ankle, or shin, or position your left foot sideways with your heel up.
- Put your hands anywhere that feels comfortable.
- Hold for one minute at most.
- Then, alternate to the opposite side.

CAT-COW STRETCH:

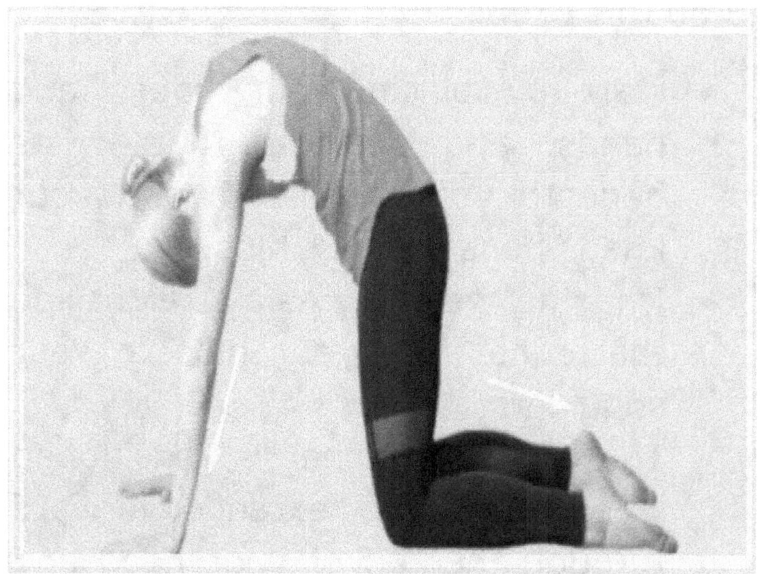

This yoga helps the back disc circulation can be enhanced by bending, stretching your spine, and improving posture and balance.

It's a simple movement, that can help you if you spend a lot of time sitting, it may be quite helpful in supporting the back, relieving discomfort, and keeping the spine healthy.

The following are the simple instructions to do this exercise:

- start by placing your knees and hands, and position your wrists beneath your shoulders and your knees beneath your hips.
- Imagine the spine as a straight line that runs from your hips to your shoulders.
- The neutral spine is positioned where the line extends forward through the top of your head and back through your tailbone.
- Maintain a long neck by looking down and out.
- Inhale and round for pose
- Twist your toes downward.
- Raise your tailbone by tilting your pelvis back.
- Allow your neck to be the final part of your spine to move, starting from your tailbone.

- Your belly falls, but bring your navel in so that your abdominal muscles embrace your spine.
- Gently raise your eyes to the ceiling without straining your neck.

DOWNWARD FACING DOG YOGA:

This yoga helps to increase the abdominal muscles, stretches the hamstring and calves, and it also strengthens the legs and arms.

In addition, this yoga helps to enhance the flow of blood from the brain when it is incorporated into your weekly activity.

The following is the instruction on how this yoga is carried out:

It is important to keep in mind that this yoga can be done anywhere with a yoga mat.

- Put your wrists under your shoulders and your knees under

your hips to perform a hands-and-knees position.

- To raise your hips and straighten your legs, tuck your toes beneath and push back through your palms.
- As you spread your fingers, grind down into your fingertips from your forearms.
- Expand the collarbones by rotating your upper arms outward.
- Lift your shoulders from your ears and toward your hips, allowing your head to dangle.
- To release the weight from your arms, firmly contract your quads. Essentially, this is a resting stance because of this movement.
- Scoop your heels down toward the ground, keep your tail up, and rotate your thighs inward.
- Verify how far apart your hands and feet are from one another.

HIGH LUNGE YOGA:

This yoga helps to strengthen your core, balance in this posture, and remain upright.

To activate your rectus abdominus and your internal and external obliques, concentrate on drawing in your navel while clutching your ribs near each other.

The following are the instructions to carry out when performing this yoga:

- First, return to the downward dog position and take five deep breaths to relax.
- Step forward your right foot in line with your right hand.
- To ensure that your right thigh is parallel to the floor, bend your right knee and position it over your right ankle.

- Take a high lunge by raising both arms toward the ceiling.
- Take five deep breaths. (Don't worry, we'll finish in a minute on the other side.)

SEATED SPINAL TWIST POSE:

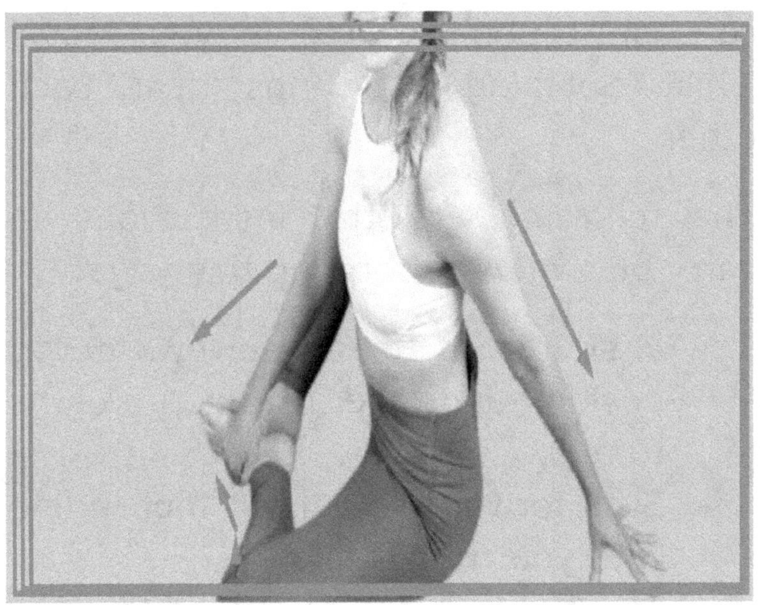

This is an excellent position to increase hip, shoulder, and spine flexibility. It helps with digestion and strengthens the lower back.

- Begin this yoga by sitting in a comfortable seated position on a yoga mat, keeping your shoulders and arms relaxed. Ensure that your legs are in a triangle form as you can see in the picture above.
- Take a deep inhalation and raise your arms. Exhale to turn to the right, placing the right hand behind the back the left hand on the right knee, and your palm holding your left leg.
- For five to ten breaths, maintain the position.
- Exhale to relax. Do the same on the opposite side.

Note that if your lower back hurts, put a folded blanket under you. Alternatively, attempt this posture as chair yoga. If necessary, seek the help of a yoga instructor.

PALM TREE YOGA POSE:

this yoga helps stretch the legs, arms, chest, belly, and spine. In addition to enhancing posture, raising awareness, and regulating breathing, it aids with attention and concentration.

This yoga also helps to improve blood circulation, aid with digestion, and strengthen your legs and abdomen, hold this posture for a longer period.

The following are the instructions to do to perform this exercise:

- Stand tall in on a yoga mat
- Take a mountain posture to begin.
- look at a particular spot. Raise your hands, clasp your fingers together above your head, and turn your palms up.
- Take a breath and raise your heels off the mat. Try to extend as much

as you can without making your back too arched.

- Take five to ten deep breaths here. Release the breath to bring the heels back to the beginning position.

TWISTING COBRA YOGA POSE:

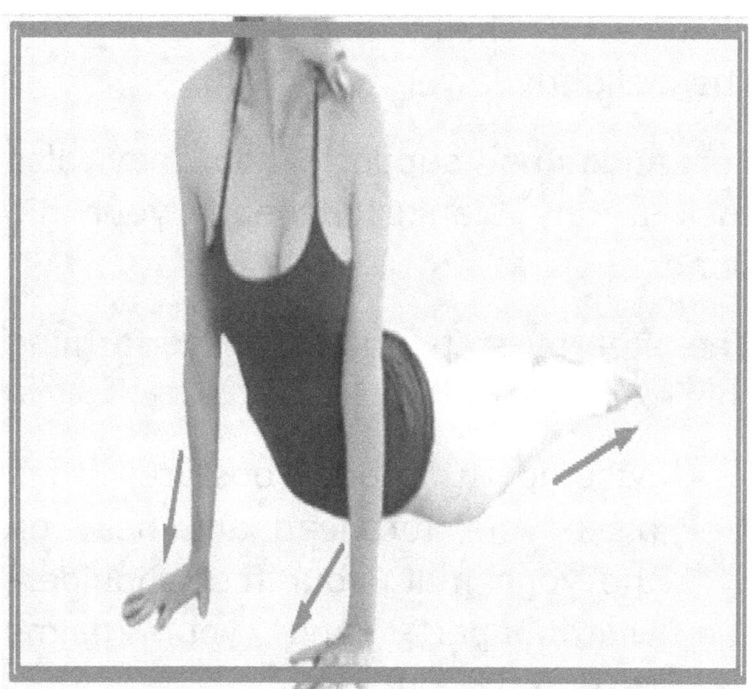

This position is excellent for improving back flexibility. It is good to incorporate into a constipation-fighting workout regimen as it stimulates and massages the kidneys and liver.

keep in mind that If you find this posture too challenging, try raising the chest slightly lower.

For additional support, you may also tuck a tiny blanket beneath your hip bones.

The step-by-step guides to performing this exercise:

- Assume a prone posture, then place your forehead and belly on the yoga mat, your feet shoulder-width apart, and your palms resting by your ribs.

- Take a breath and raise your head and chest until your arms are straight. Refrain from slapping shoulders.
- To turn to the right, exhale. Take three to five breaths here.
- Breathe in to return to the centre, then out to descend again. Continue on the opposite side.

CORPSE YOGA POSE:

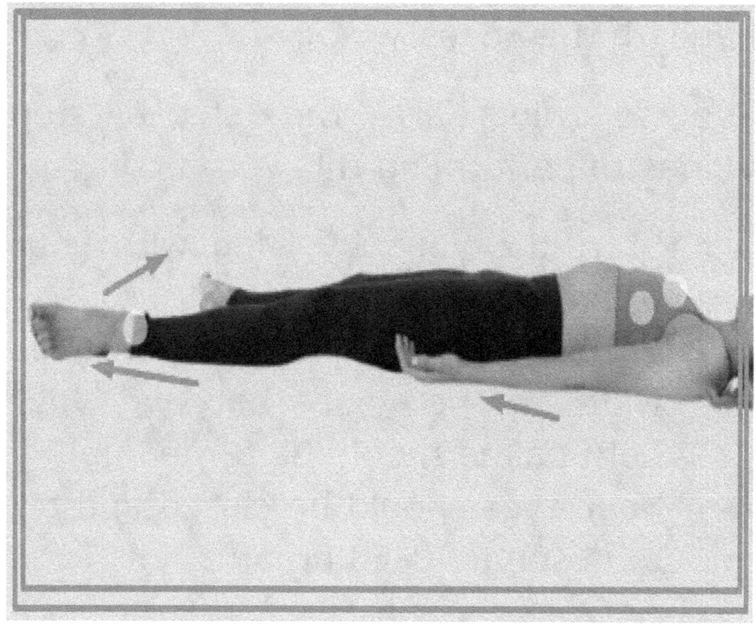

This yoga stance, which helps relax the body and quiet the mind, is perhaps one of the most crucial poses in a yoga practice.

Since it takes a lot of effort to still the mind, this is one of the most difficult yoga postures for a Hatha or restorative yoga teacher to teach.

Note that if you are suffering from back ache it is important to Put a cushion beneath the knees.

The following are the step-by-step guides to performing this yoga:

- Start the yoga by lying with your back flat on the yoga mat.
- Ensure you spread your feet as wide as the yoga mat and your both palms should be turned up.
- Your eyes should be closed and try to observe 20-50 breaths.

- Start with little motions around the fingers and toes, then work your way up to the remainder of the body to relax.

CHAPTER 6: PILATE WORKOUTS TO IMPROVE CORE STABILITY AND BALANCE AND ENHANCE POSTURAL ALIGNMENT.

Pilates workouts are known for targeting stability and strength in the core. Pilate workouts can be used to target postural alignment in the body, improve balance, and prevent injury in seniors.

It is very important to note that most pilates are very easy to perform. For this reason, every senior should try to incorporate Pilates exercises into their daily exercises.

in this chapter, please keep in mind that we are going to be performing simple pilates exercises that can help to improve core stability, and balance and enhance postural alignment.

However, ensure that you grab your mat, and your exercise wears and also create a space as we work you through this simple pilates:

The following are the pilate workouts for seniors:

SIDE LEG LIFT PILATE:

This pilate helps to strengthen the abdominal muscles, the back, and the inner tight.

This pilate aims to Maintain your body in a straight line can help you stay in alignment. Check your ribs and lower back to make sure you're not overarching.

The following are how to perform this pilate:

- With your legs straight and parallel to your hips, lie on your side. Place your ear on your lower arm while keeping it extended overhead. For balance, place the upper arm's hand on the ground in front of your lower abdomen.

- Exhale to raise both legs off the ground and stretch your upper body and legs in opposition.
- Control your breathing to bring your legs down.
- After 8–10 repetitions, switch sides.

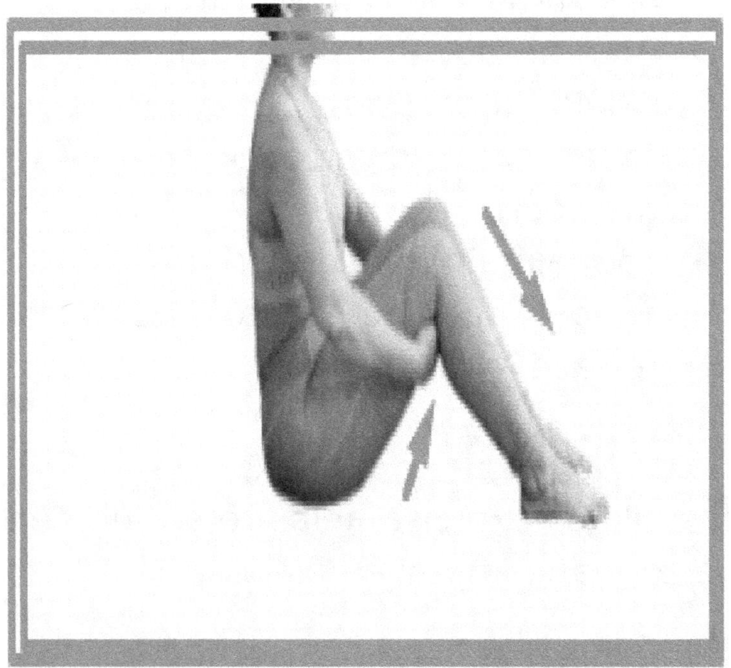

This pilate helps to strengthen the abdominal, and back extensor muscles.

The following are how to perform this pilate:

- With your feet flat on the floor and your knees bent, take a tall seat to start. You can put your hands lightly on the backs of your thighs or extend your arms forward.

- Breathe out to bring your abs and pelvic floor inward. Tilt your pelvis to curl your lower back halfway to the floor.
- To maintain the curl, inhale.
- To get back to where you were, release the breath.

PENDULUM PILATE:

This pilates exercise helps to strengthen the core and improve balance.

The following are how to perform it effectively:

- With your arms out to your sides, lie face up. Lift your feet off the mat and bend your knees over your hips.
- Maintaining your lower back on the floor, let both knees drop to the right.

- Go back to the beginning and repeat the process on the opposite side.

LEGS CIRCLE PILATE:

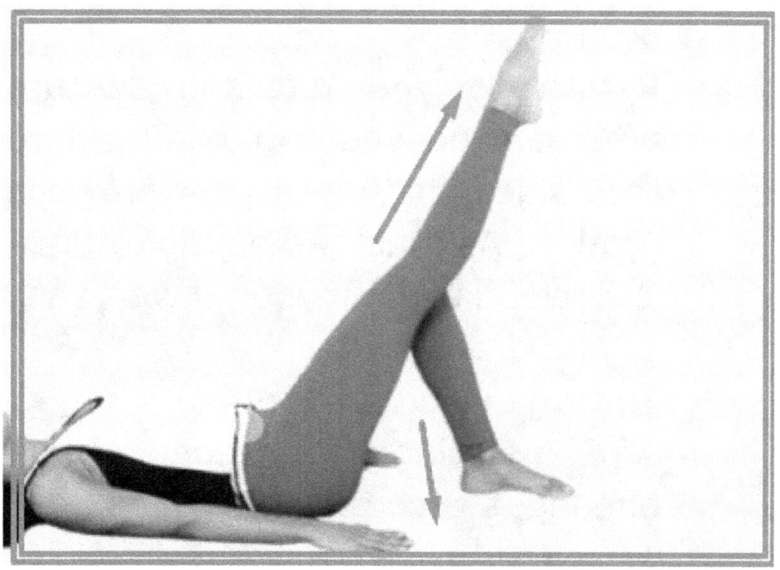

This pilate helps to improve stability and balance, and strengthen the muscles in the lower body.

The following are how to perform this pilate:

- With your arms at your sides and your palms down, lie and face up.
- With your left foot flat on the ground, bend your left knee. Raise your right leg till it is parallel to the ground.
- Return to your starting posture after circling your right leg out to the side and down toward the ground. As much as possible, draw a circle, keeping your lower back on the ground.
- Turn the circle around.
- After finishing each repetition on one leg, switch to the other.

GET IN MOTION:

This pilate helps to strengthen the core both the upper and the lower parts of the body.

The following are how to perform this pilate:

- Arms stretched over your head, lying on the floor, while you lie face up.
- Raise your arms to the point where your wrists meet your shoulders, and then slowly curl your spine off the ground, beginning at your shoulders and working your way down to your lower back.
- Maintaining a taut core throughout, curl up into a sitting posture and then continue folding your torso over your legs.
- Roll back down to the floor by reversing the motion and lowering your shoulders to your lower back.

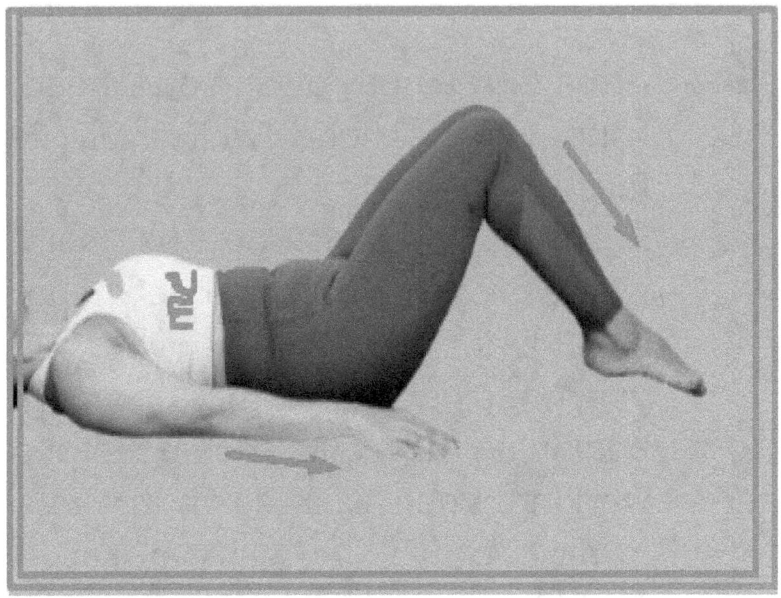

To perform this pilate the following are the steps to take:

- With your feet flat on the ground and your arms by your sides, lie on your back on a mat. Ensure that your back is flat on the mat.
- Raise your knees to about a 90-degree position. This is the initial position.

- Bring your feet down slowly enough for your toes to tap the floor. To get back to where you were before, reverse the motion. This counts as one rep.

SWAN DIVE PILATE:

This exercise helps to strengthen the muscles in the abdominal, back, and hip extensors.

How to perform this exercise:

- To start this exercise, lie and face down on the floor, place your hands flat and parallel to your shoulders while maintaining a bent elbow position.
- With your body in an active position, your lower back extended (avoid sinking or arching into your lower back), and your abs pulled in and up. Your hamstrings and

glutes are working when your legs are extended and straight.

- Inhale to picture reaching through the top of your head. As far as your body will allow without straining, raise your head, chest, and ribs while gently pressing into the floor with your hands.
- Take a breath out to expand your torso and get back on the mat.
- Repeat 5-8 times.